Frequently Asked Questions

all about
chromium picolinate

GARY EVANS, PhD

AVERY PUBLISHING GROUP

Garden City Park • New York

The information contained in this book is based upon the research and personal and professional experiences of the author. It is not intended as a substitute for consulting with your physician or other health care provider. Any attempt to diagnose and treat an illness should be done under the direction of a health care professional.

The publisher does not advocate the use of any particular health care protocol, but believes the information in this book should be available to the public. The publisher and author are not responsible for any adverse effects or consequences resulting from the use of any of the suggestions, preparations, or procedures discussed in this book. Should the reader have any questions concerning the appropriateness of any procedure or preparation mentioned, the author and the publisher strongly suggest consulting a professional health care advisor.

Series cover designer: Eric Macaluso
Cover image courtesy of Steven Foster Group, Inc.

Avery Publishing Group, Inc.
120 Old Broadway, Garden City Park, NY 11040
1-800-548-5757 or visit us at www.averypublishing.com

ISBN: 0-89529-876-7

Printed in the United States of America

10   9   8   7   6   5   4   3   2

Contents

Introduction

Can a nutrient that you need in infinitesimal amounts be a major influence on your health and well-being? Yes, if that mineral is chromium, of which most people need only 200 mcg—an incredibly miniscule fraction of an ounce—on a daily basis.

Chromium was first recognized as an important dietary mineral some forty years ago. However, it remained relatively unknown to the general public until a particular form of chromium, called chromium picolinate, was discovered.

How does this simple dietary mineral affect your health, you ask? Chromium works in large part by improving the efficiency of insulin, a hormone that orchestrates the movement of sugar and fat into your body's cells, where they are either burned for fuel or stored for later use. To do its work, insulin depends on chromium, and when levels of this mineral are low, insulin cannot perform as it should. The consequence can set the stage for obesity, heart disease, and diabetes.

Because chromium picolinate enables insulin to

work better, diabetics who take this remarkable supplement have a much easier time controlling some of the complications associated with their disease. Several clinical studies have shown that chromium improves insulin activity in diabetics. In fact, studies with many different kinds of animals have shown that half as much insulin is needed by the body for it to perform its functions when chromium picolinate is added to the diet—another sign that chromium improves insulin activity.

You don't have to be a diabetic, however, to benefit from chromium picolinate. This mineral has other benefits as well. For example, you have probably heard of LDL and HDL cholesterol. LDL, or low-density lipoprotein, is the so-called bad cholesterol strongly associated with heart-disease risk. HDL, or high-density lipoprotein, is the good cholesterol that seems to protect against heart disease. Scientific studies have shown that taking chromium-picolinate supplements decreases total cholesterol and LDL-cholesterol levels, while increasing HDL-cholesterol levels.

Studies have also shown that exercising regularly coupled with taking chromium-picolinate supplements produces a dramatic increase in muscle mass along with a marked reduction in body fat. Many body builders swear by chromium picolinate. One study even found that non-exercising individuals had a pronounced loss of body fat (and no loss of muscle) after taking chromium-picolinate supplements for just three months.

Since chromium picolinate was discovered, a great deal of sound scientific data has been accumulated supporting its safety and health benefits. There has also been a great deal of misinformation printed and spoken about chromium picolinate, mostly by people who have never bothered to look at the dozens of studies that show the benefits of this form of chromium. *All About Chromium Picolinate* should help you to understand the importance of this research.

1.

Why You Need
Chromium Picolinate

Chromium is a mineral your body needs for the hormone insulin to work efficiently and effectively. Unfortunately, chromium is difficult to get from the diet because many processed foods lack it. Chromium-picolinate supplements usually contain enough chromium to satisfy the needs of the body in a form your cells can assimilate and use.

Q. What's the relationship between chromium and insulin?

A. Your body secretes insulin after you eat. Insulin is a hormone, a compound that regulates many body processes. Insulin's primary purpose is to transport glucose, also known as blood sugar, from the blood to the cells of your body. In the cells, glucose is a fuel, much like the gasoline you add to your car. Without glucose, your body's 100 trillion cells cannot function. Basically, insulin makes it possible for the glucose to get into your cells and to power up the cells' energy levels.

Without sufficient chromium, insulin cannot function optimally and your body cannot properly manage the breakdown of glucose and fats. Because of its central role in the utilization of digested food, chromium is one of the most important minerals in the body. Unfortunately, it is also one of the most difficult to obtain from food. Soil levels of chromium are often poor, so food levels are often limited as well. In addition, processing frequently removes this mineral from food.

Q. Is there a disease caused by not getting enough chromium?

A. A lack of chromium appears to increase the risk of insulin resistance, a condition also called syndrome X. This disorder is characterized by high levels of insulin and glucose. Basically, in syndrome X, the body cannot properly process glucose, so it secretes more and more insulin. Unfortunately, the insulin does not work very efficiently, a situation due in part to the lack of chromium.

This is significant because syndrome X is strongly associated with elevated levels of cholesterol and other blood fats, and an increased risk of heart disease and diabetes. An estimated 20 to 25 percent of the population suffers from syndrome X, with most cases undiagnosed.

Q. What are the best sources of chromium?

A. Unfortunately, no particular food group can be singled out as a good source of chromium. For example, dairy products generally have less than 1 mcg of chromium per serving. Meats, poultry, and fish are a little better, with 1 to 10 mcg per serving. Grain products, including whole-grain breads, don't provide more than 8 mcg per serving. Fruits and vegetables, generally good sources of nutrients, don't have much more than a few micrograms of chromium per serving. The one exception in this last food group is broccoli, which contains more than 20 mcg of chromium in a serving.

A few years ago, Richard Anderson, Ph.D., along with an associate at the U.S. Department of Agriculture (USDA) published a paper showing how inadequate our diets are in terms of chromium. These USDA scientists measured the daily intake of chromium by thirty-two men and women for seven days. These people were asked to eat just as they would if not participating in a study. It turned out that nobody in the study consumed more than 33 mcg of chromium per day over the seven-day period. This amount is well below the National Academy of Sciences' recommendation of 50 mcg per day and the Food and Drug Administration's reference daily intake of 130 mcg.

Dietary analyses show there are, on average, about 14 mcg of chromium in every 1,000 calories of food. Based on this, you would have to eat more than 14,000 calories daily to consume sufficient chromium. As a consequence, it is not unreasonable to recommend that people supplement their diets with chromium picolinate.

Q. What exactly is chromium picolinate?

A. Chromium picolinate is a combination of the essential mineral chromium and the little-known chemical picolinate, which is made from a natural substance called picolinic acid. This compound promotes efficient chromium absorption.

The minerals you need in your body are in a form called ions. An ion is the electrically charged version of a mineral. Chromium is a supercharged ion, and it has to be deenergized before your body's cells will allow it to approach and enter. The membrane "fence" that surrounds the cells repels anything that is charged, so ions have to first be deactivated. Chromium accomplishes this by attaching to special chemical substances called chelators, which deactivate ions. Gary Evans, Ph.D., a USDA researcher, discovered picolinate to be a superior chelator and showed that it very effectively cloaks the charge of chromium, enabling the mineral to be carried by the blood to the cells that need it.

Q. Are there any natural sources of chromium picolinate?

A. The natural sources of chromium picolinate include brewer's yeast, liver, and kidney. But unless you eat copious amounts of these foods—some of which are not very appetizing—chromium picolinate is nearly impossible to get from the diet without daily supplementation. A person would have to consume about a quarter of a pound of brewer's yeast, liver, or kidney on a daily basis to get adequate amounts of chromium picolinate from natural sources. Even beer, which is made with brewer's yeast, doesn't have much more than 50 mcg in a 1-lit pitcher. Needless to say, no dietitian or nutritionist would ever recommend drinking four to six pitchers of beer a day to meet your chromium requirement.

Q. When should people start taking chromium-picolinate supplements?

A. Years ago, Henry Schroeder, Ph.D., one of the pioneers in chromium research, showed that the chromium level in the body is highest right after birth, then decreases with age. Studies with pigs, rats, rabbits, and chickens also demonstrated that the chromium level becomes less than adequate soon after birth. As the chromium level declines in the body, insulin becomes less effective, increasing the risk of abnormalities in all the insulin-dependent systems in the body. Beginning chromium-picolinate supplementation in childhood would therefore be beneficial.

While taking chromium-picolinate supplements is a smart move for all adults, if you eat a lot of sugary foods and refined carbohydrates, such as sweets, pasta, and white bread, it is especially important. This is because the effectiveness of insulin in the body decreases when you eat high amounts of these foods. When you consume too much sugar, your muscle cells temporarily switch off their insulin-recognition system, redirecting the glucose to your fat stores and your liver. Ultimately, the fat cells stop recognizing insulin and start ignoring it—that is, they become insulin resistant. This is followed by an almost total closing down of the biological systems that shuttle glucose into the muscle cells and fat cells. When insulin can no longer stimulate these cells to pull the glucose out of the blood, the glucose spills into the urine. This is a characteristic sign of diabetes. It is important, however, to point out that a person can have trouble with insulin and insulin resistance (syndrome X) without being diabetic.

Q. What is the difference between chromium picolinate and chromium polynicotinate?

A. Chromium picolinate is chromium chemically combined with picolinate to make a nutrient the body can use. Chromium polynicotinate is merely a mixture of chromium and nicotinate (a form of vitamin B_3) combined with water. Picolinate and nicotinate are what chemists call isomers—that is, they have the same atoms, but in different arrangements and with different chemical properties. The atoms in picolinate are arranged in a way that make the substance an ideal metal chelator. The atoms in nicotinate have a different arrangement, and the resulting substance is not a good metal ion chelator.

Since nicotinate is an isomer of picolinate, the manufacturers of chromium polynicotinate assumed and advertised that the supplement was also a chelated form of chromium. However, according to a study published in the *Journal of Inorganic Biochemistry*, scientists at the USDA determined the exact chemical forms of chromium polynicotinate and chromium picolinate, and found that only chromium picolinate is a chelator. Chromium picolinate was determined to be a chelate made of chromium attached to three picolinate molecules, a finding in complete agreement with other studies. Chromium polynicotinate was not determined to be a chelated form of chromium. These differences affect how well chromium is absorbed by the body.

Q. How much chromium does a person need?

A. The amount of chromium a person needs depends upon his or her age, daily activity level, and overall health. For example, teenaged boys might benefit from 300 to 400 mcg daily, whereas teenaged girls might benefit from 200 to 300 mcg.

Of course, it's always best to discuss your individual requirement with a nutritionally oriented physician, particularly if you're a parent planning supplementation for a child. Adults up to retirement age would be well advised to use a daily supplement supplying 400 mcg of chromium. Elderly people should take at least 200 mcg. Some studies have found that diabetics can benefit from a daily intake of 1,000 mcg of chromium as chromium picolinate. However, they must be watchful for decreases in their insulin or hypoglycemic-medication requirements.

Keep in mind that these dosage suggestions are very general. If you are very active or, conversely, engage in very little physical exercise, you may want to adjust your chromium intake to coincide more closely with the number of calories you consume per day. Close scrutiny of all the studies using either humans or animals shows that the most dramatic and consistent results were obtained when the daily supplement contained at least 200 mcg of chromium as picolinate for every 1,000 calories of food eaten. Thus, if you eat 2,000 calories daily, you might do best with 400 mcg of chromium as picolinate.

These rough chromium requirement estimates are based on research work done with chromium picolinate in both humans and animals. However, there are two very important points to keep in mind when considering them. First, these recommendations assume that you will be using chromium picolinate rather than some other, less effective form. Second, the quantities listed in these recommendations are for chromium, not for the entire chemical complex of chromium picolinate.

Q. How much chromium is included in chromium picolinate?

A. Chromium picolinate is a complex chemical, and pure elemental chromium makes up only 12 percent of the whole unit. Unfortunately, some manufacturers have confusing wording on the labels of their supplement bottles. For example, a supplement that, according to the label, contains 500 mcg of chromium picolinate actually has only 60 mcg of elemental chromium. You would have to take at least seven of these capsules every day to receive any benefits. The labels on chromium-picolinate supplement bottles should state how many micrograms of pure elemental chromium are contained in each capsule, as well as how many total micrograms of chromium picolinate there are. Always read the ingredients label to determine if the supplement has the proper amount of chromium, and ask questions if the label is not clear.

Q. Do the other forms of chromium work like chromium picolinate?

A. Dr. Anderson and his associates at the USDA investigated some of the chromium chelators by putting a variety of the different kinds of chromium into the diets of laboratory rats. They found that the amount of chromium in the liver was the greatest in the rats fed chromium picolinate. In contrast, the amount of chromium in the livers of the rats fed chromium polynicotinate was the same as the amount of chromium in the livers of the rats given no chromium at all! Also, the amount of chromium in the kidneys and spleens of the rats fed chromium picolinate was greater than the amount of chromium in the kidneys and spleens of the rats fed chromium polynicotinate.

In a human study, Dr. Anderson and his associates administered daily supplements of the different kinds of chromium. By measuring the amount of chromium in the blood and urine, they discovered that chromium picolinate was the only form of chromium absorbed efficiently by the humans. This study convinced Dr. Anderson to use chromium picolinate in a much publicized study with type-II diabetics that produced spectacular results. (This study is described in Chapter 2.)

Several other studies with both humans and animals demonstrated that the type of chromium used in a supplement does make a difference in how the supplement is absorbed. In one study, Dr. Evans and his students at Bimidji State University in Minnesota fed rats chromium picolinate, chromium polynicotinate, and chromium chloride. They found that the rats given chromium picolinate had lower blood-glucose levels and lived much longer than the rats fed the other forms of chromium. In fact, the most ineffective type of chromium supplement appeared to be chromium chloride, which is the form often found in multimineral supplements.

Q. Is it necessary to have your blood checked to determine if you need to take chromium-picolinate supplements?

A. Unfortunately, blood-chromium analyses are currently difficult and expensive, and, as a result, are not commonly performed. Hair analysis is another method to measure the levels of chromium and other minerals in the body. The theory is that the hair level of a mineral reflects the level of that mineral in the other tissues in the body. Most nutritionally oriented physicians can arrange for you to have your hair analyzed.

There is another way to determine whether your insulin is working properly—the glucose tolerance test. You may want to take this test if you have a strong family history of diabetes; if you have problems with mood swings or food cravings; or if you have any of the symptoms of diabetes, such as unusual thirst, frequent urination, unexplained weight loss, or drowsiness. You will be asked not to eat anything for twelve hours before taking the test. At the start of the test, a small amount of blood will be taken from your fingertip to obtain a baseline for comparisons. Next, you will be given a drink that contains glucose. After that, blood will be drawn over a period of a few hours. These blood samples will allow your doctor to see how quickly your body removes glucose from your bloodstream. The time it takes for your blood-glucose level to rise and then return to the baseline level will tell your doctor whether or not your insulin is working as it should.

Without a test, though, it may be fair to assume that, because of the standard American diet, you don't have enough chromium in your body to keep your insulin working at maximum efficiency. I often recommend that my patients test themselves for thirty days with nutritional supplements. So, I suggest that you try taking chromium picolinate for thirty days to see if you feel better. If you don't notice a change after this amount of time, stop taking the chromium. You may find, however, that you feel better taking the chromium picolinate than not taking it.

2.

Chromium Picolinate and Diabetes

Many scientific studies have shown that chromium picolinate enables insulin to work much more efficiently. Because of its action on this important hormone, chromium is a key nutrient in the prevention and control of diabetes.

Q. What is diabetes?

A. Diabetes is a defect in how the body uses insulin to metabolize glucose. There are two principal types of diabetes. One is called type-I, juvenile-onset, or insulin-dependent diabetes. This type affects about 1 million Americans and generally develops during childhood. People lose the ability to produce insulin, and so they must have insulin shots on a daily basis.

The other type of diabetes is called type-II, adult-onset, or noninsulin-dependent diabetes. This type of diabetes is caused by an overproduction of insulin or insulin resistance. Type-II diabetes typically affects adults, although overweight children can also develop it. It affects 10 million to 15 million Americans, and can generally be controlled by diet, weight loss, and hypoglycemic (blood-glucose-lowering) drugs. However, chromium picolinate can help many aspects of type-II diabetes because it improves the efficiency of insulin.

Q. Can chromium picolinate help type-I diabetics who must inject insulin?

A. Chromium picolinate can help type-I diabetics by making their injected insulin more effective. Before insulin was discovered, diabetics wasted away and died because their cells were unable to absorb glucose. Now, insulin is readily available, so diabetics can start giving themselves insulin injections as soon as their disease is diagnosed. The daily injections must be continued through life, however. Unfortunately, injected insulin is not completely effective. As a result, blood glucose is not always adequately controlled, resulting sometimes in too much glucose and too much insulin (the injected kind) present at the same time.

Insulin triggers a number of chemical reactions

that cause fat to be deposited in the adipose (fat) cells, whereas high blood-glucose levels turn off the mechanism that releases fat from these cells. Soon after diabetics start injecting insulin, they often have difficulty controlling their body fat. Increased body fat is one of the many problems caused by having too much insulin and too much glucose in the blood at the same time.

In animal studies, scientists showed that chromium-picolinate supplements led to normal or more rapid clearance of glucose from the blood with much less insulin. This is a sign of efficient insulin action. Many investigators have noted a marked improvement in insulin action when chromium is added in test-tube experiments. Some research has indicated that type-I diabetics can reduce the amount of insulin they need by taking chromium-picolinate supplements.

However, and this is *very* important: Type-I diabetics who take chromium picolinate must monitor their blood-glucose levels very carefully. Chromium picolinate increases the efficiency of injected insulin, which could lead to hypoglycemic shock (from taking too much insulin). If you are a diabetic taking insulin, discuss your chromium-picolinate dosage with your physician. Long-term, chromium-picolinate supplements should assist your insulin injections in stabilizing your glucose level.

Q. How does chromium picolinate help people with type-II diabetes?

A. The benefits of chromium picolinate in type-II diabetes have been demonstrated in both human and animal studies. William Cefalu, M.D., director of the Diabetes Comprehensive Care and Research Program at the Bowman Gray School of Medicine, Winston-Salem, North Carolina, recently presented the results of a human trial with chromium picolinate at a meeting of the American Diabetes Association. Overweight individuals with family histories of diabetes were given 1,000 mcg of chromium as chromium picolinate daily. After four months, their insulin resistance was reduced markedly, and the improvement continued until the end of the study at eight months.

Dr. Cefalu noted: "Even though only a small number of subjects were studied, the improvement in insulin sensitivity in chromium-supplemented subjects was quite significant and impressive. This is a potentially important finding in light of the fact that insulin resistance often precedes Type II diabetes. Chromium picolinate is a nutritional supplement that can reduce risk factors for the development of diabetes."

At the 56th Annual Scientific Session of the

American Diabetes Association in 1996, Dr. Richard Anderson described the results of a study involving 180 Chinese subjects who had been diagnosed with type-II diabetes. Anderson described the results as "spectacular!" Prior to the studies conducted by Drs. Cefalu and Anderson, several clinical trials had shown that chromium supplements in the form of chromium picolinate helped to control the levels of blood glucose and blood fats, including cholesterol. Moreover, several studies conducted with animals, particularly swine, had shown that chromium-picolinate supplements markedly improved insulin action, leading to an improved control of blood glucose, blood fats, and body fat.

The same as type-I diabetics, type-II diabetics who take chromium picolinate need to carefully monitor their blood-glucose levels. This is especially true if you take a hypoglycemic medication to lower your blood-glucose level. Again, chromium picolinate increases the efficiency of injected insulin and hypoglycemic medications.

Q. What about taking chromium picolinate for gestational diabetes?

A. Chromium picolinate has been shown to possibly reduce the risk of gestational diabetes, a temporary diabetic condition that often occurs during pregnancy, and it also appears to be safe. However, most of the evidence here is based on animal studies.

Studies with pigs provided good evidence that chromium picolinate is a safe supplement to use during pregnancy. Dr. Merlin Lindemann and his associates showed that chromium picolinate slowed fat development and improved insulin action in pigs, and also had other important benefits. Dr. Lindemann's team fed female pigs chromium picolinate beginning when they were gilts (very young) through the time they delivered two litters. The sows fed chromium picolinate for more than nine months used 27-percent less insulin than the gilts fed chromium picolinate for thirty-five days to clear blood glucose. The sows given no chromium supplements used 45-percent more insulin than the gilts to clear blood glucose. The sows fed chromium picolinate used less than half as much insulin to clear blood glucose as the sows given no supplements. Without chromium-picolinate supplementation, the pigs' insulin efficiency steadily eroded as the animals matured.

Furthermore, the litter weight of the pigs from the supplemented sows was 26-percent greater at birth and 22-percent greater after twenty-one days. Of the eleven sows that were not given chromium picolinate, only six (55 percent) had a second litter.

However, ten of the eleven sows (91 percent) given chromium picolinate had second litters. Similar positive trends have been found in other studies.

Chromium-picolinate supplements obviously caused no problems in experimental animals during pregnancy and thus should be safe for humans, since the physiologies of humans and pigs are similar. Dr. Lois Jovanovic of the Samsum Medical Research Foundation in Santa Clara, California, has done clinical studies with chromium picolinate in pregnant women, and she recommends chromium picolinate to prevent the occurrence of gestational diabetes.

Q. What other benefits can chromium picolinate provide type-II diabetics?

A. Two very comprehensive studies led by Dr. Anderson demonstrated a number of other benefits provided by chromium-picolinate supplementation. In the first study, type-II diabetics taking some type of medication were given either 200 mcg or 1,000 mcg of chromium daily as chromium picolinate. Their blood glucose, insulin, cholesterol, and hemoglobin A1C, an indicator of diabetic control, were all improved. The subjects who were given 1,000 mcg of chromium per day benefited the most because diabetics have an increased need for chromium.

In the second study, which was designed to determine whether the benefits of taking chromium-picolinate supplements persisted, more than 800 people were studied for a period of ten months. Their blood-glucose levels decreased during the first month and remained lower for the following nine months. The symptoms of diabetes, including fatigue, thirst, and frequent urination, decreased dramatically during the first month and continued to be less throughout the ten-month study. During this study, all the subjects took glucose-lowering medications along with 1,000 mcg of chromium as chromium picolinate.

Q. So, you're *not* recommending that diabetics stop taking their medications, right?

A. No one should ever stop taking a prescribed medication without consulting with a physician. The studies conducted by Dr. Anderson and his colleagues, as well as several other clinical trials, all showed that chromium, particularly when given as chromium picolinate, was very helpful in the treatment of type-II diabetes. It was not given in place of any medications, however. Again, diabetics who take chromium picolinate need to monitor their blood-glucose levels *very* carefully. A sudden improvement in how the body uses insulin could decrease the medication requirements, which could, in effect, lead to a sudden drug overdose.

Q. Can chromium picolinate be used in place of insulin?

A. The same as in type-II diabetes, chromium picolinate works with insulin in type-I diabetes, but it does not replace insulin or mimic insulin's activities. Insulin is a protein, made from amino acids, and is secreted from the pancreas. Its job is to direct glucose, amino acids, and fat into the cells. Whether chromium interacts with insulin directly, with insulin's target cells, or both, insulin is much more effective when chromium is present. Because insulin needs chromium for optimal action, chromium picolinate is a cofactor for insulin.

Q. Does chromium picolinate help hypoglycemia?

A. It depends on the type of hypoglycemia. Hypoglycemia means low blood glucose ("hypo" means "low," "glyc" means "glucose," and "emia" means "blood"). True hypoglycemia is a chronic (long-term) condition in which the body has a difficult time keeping the blood-glucose level high enough for normal brain function. This particular problem is caused by the inability of the body to make a hormone called glucagon. Glucagon is released from special cells in the pancreas when those cells sense that the level of blood glucose is too low to keep the brain functioning as it should. Glucagon stimulates the liver to release glucose into the blood so that the blood glucose will return to a level sufficient to satisfy the brain's requirements. A person who cannot make glucagon for the purpose of keeping a normal blood-glucose level must have the condition treated by a physician. Chromium picolinate would not be of help to a person who does not make sufficient glucagon.

Q. What about reactive hypoglycemia?

A. Chromium-picolinate supplements may be helpful to people with reactive hypoglycemia. Reactive hypoglycemia, the kind that occurs most often, is a condition in which ineffective insulin causes the blood-glucose level to build up and then suddenly to drop below what is considered normal. In a sense, it is a type of hypoglycemia caused in reaction to a meal, especially a high-sugar meal. A person who has reactive hypoglycemia often goes from feeling anxious and hyperactive to feeling listless and depressed. The problem is characterized by mood swings and food cravings. Reactive hypoglycemia often precedes the development of insulin resistance. The condition should be considered as a warning that insulin is not functioning properly in the body.

Q. What does chromium picolinate do to make insulin work better?

A. To the best of our knowledge, chromium picolinate most likely combines with insulin to make it act more effectively. One of insulin's many jobs is to stimulate the body's muscle and fat cells to remove glucose from the blood. It does this by first hooking onto a specialized chemical on the cell called a receptor. This receptor then sends a message to the inside of the cell calling for glucose movers to go to the blood, pick up the glucose, and transport it to the inside of the cell. Before any signal can be sent to the cell's interior, however, the insulin must reach the receptor and become attached. To get to the cell, the insulin must float through the blood until it reaches the blood capillary next to its destination. It then must pass through the walls of the capillary. The more efficient the insulin is, the easier it will be for the glucose to pass through the capillary walls.

Once the insulin reaches the fluid in the harbor around the cell, it has to move into its designated molecular dock. If it's too big, it will scrape the sides of the protein pier, making mooring difficult. If it's too small, it might be tossed around in the fluid around the cell, also making mooring difficult. Insulin must be a prescribed size and shape so that it can slip through the capillary and slide into port. When insulin fails to move easily from the blood or dock, it can't stimulate glucose clearance. Chromium may play a role in keeping insulin just the right shape so that it can maneuver through the capillary walls and fit into the chemical ports designed to hold it.

Q. What is the difference between chromium picolinate and vanadyl sulfate?

A. Chromium picolinate makes insulin work more effectively, whereas vanadyl sulfate actually mimics the action of insulin. Vanadyl sulfate is a chemical compound made of vanadium, a mineral, and sulfate, a complex of sulfur and oxygen. Several years ago, a Canadian scientist discovered that vanadyl sulfate and other chemicals that contain vanadium affect the cells in much the same way as insulin. The scientist's original intention was to use vanadyl sulfate to learn how insulin works in the cells. Because vanadyl sulfate acts like insulin, and many experts think of insulin as an anabolic (muscle-building) hormone, many athletes and body builders began using the supplement to help develop their muscles.

However, because vanadyl sulfate mimics the action of insulin, there is a potential problem that could arise in persons who use the compound as a supplement. While taking vanadyl-sulfate supplements, your need for naturally produced insulin decreases. Vanadium may turn off the pancreatic cells that make insulin, and when you stop taking vanadium, your body may not produce enough insulin for a while. You will, in effect, be diabetic until your cells become completely rejuvenated.

3.

Chromium Picolinate and Fat

Insulin plays an important role in determining what happens to the end products of the food you eat. Chromium picolinate is very useful in helping to control body fat because it keeps insulin working efficiently.

Q. Does chromium picolinate really melt fat?

A. By itself, chromium picolinate does nothing, and it certainly doesn't melt fat. We eat food primarily to get fuel to keep our bodies working. This fuel comes in the forms of sugars (carbohydrates) and fats. If everything works correctly, the fuel is burned and not stored, at least not for long periods. Our bodies need to maintain a constant temperature to work properly, so the cells burn fat to produce body heat. This process is called thermogenesis. In addition, many organs are constantly at work. The sum of these background activities is called the basal metabolic rate (BMR). Together, thermogenesis and the BMR burn nearly 75 percent of the body's fuel. When these two processes work optimally, there's not much fuel left to be stored. However, neither process works effectively unless insulin is present and efficient.

Insulin determines whether fat can enter the muscles, where it is used for energy. The fat stored inside adipose cells is hooked to a chemical called glycerol. Glycerol holds three strings of fat, called triglycerides. The breakdown, or so-called melting, of this fat produces energy. Before this fat can be used for fuel, however, the fats in the triglyceride strings have to be unhooked one at a time so that they can be attached to albumin, a protein in blood, and carried to the muscles. The fats are detached by enzymes that are turned on only when the blood-glucose level drops. Since the blood-glucose level doesn't drop unless insulin reaches the cells to summon the glucose movers, these enzymes don't see much action. Fat moves in easily, but gets trapped when insulin doesn't work.

When insulin doesn't do its job correctly, it is very difficult to control body composition. Thermogenesis doesn't work efficiently, the BMR is sluggish, and the fat can't get from its storehouse to the furnaces where it should be burned. Chromium picolinate keeps insulin functioning effectively, and more efficient insulin action in turn keeps the fat-burning mechanisms operating optimally.

Q. Does chromium picolinate help to stop the production of fat?

A. Chromium-picolinate supplements make insulin work more effectively, which in turn helps the body to use fat as a source of fuel to power the muscles. Insulin, and thus chromium picolinate, also influences fat production through the hormone dehydroepiandrosterone (DHEA).

The enzyme that starts the conversion of glucose into fat inside the adipose cells is switched off by DHEA. When DHEA is abundant, fat production is limited. However, when DHEA is not being synthesized, fat production in the adipose cells goes on unabated because there is no hormone to switch off the enzyme that starts the conversion of glucose to fat.

Without enough chromium in the body, insulin becomes much less efficient. The body must produce more insulin to enable the hormone to accomplish its purpose. As it turns out, too much insulin turns off the DHEA-manufacturing process. By helping to keep insulin working properly, chromium-picolinate supplements prevent the insulin levels from rising too high and blocking the production of DHEA, the hormone that stops fat production.

Q. Do you need to cut calories when using chromium picolinate to lose fat?

A. Several clinical studies have found that while using chromium-picolinate supplements, it is not necessary to drastically cut your calories to lose fat. In fact, severely cutting your food intake (unless you're seriously obese) can be harmful because it leads to muscle breakdown. Gil Kaats, Ph.D., and a team of doctors specializing in psychology, anatomical pathology, bariatric medicine, and internal medicine in San Antonio, Texas, conducted studies that showed chromium picolinate, either separately or in conjunction with other supplements and diet management, is very effective at bringing about a loss of body fat without a drastic cut in caloric intake.

In one study, the use of chromium-picolinate supplements—with no other dietary alterations—resulted in a loss of about 0.5 lb of body fat per week in obese people. At that rate, it would take six months to lose 13 lb of fat. However, a second study led by Dr. Kaats showed that people who increased their fiber intake (for example, by eating more fruits, vegetables, and grains), moderately restricted their caloric intake, and took 200 mg of carnitine and 400 to 600 mcg of chromium picolinate daily lost 12 lb of body fat in only two months. Dr. Kaats' research also showed that people can lose 12 lb of body fat in ten weeks by sticking with their current diet (assuming it has less than 25 to 40 percent of calories from fat), exercising moderately, and taking 400 to 600 mcg of chromium per day. These goals can be accomplished without a loss in muscle mass or energy, which too often occurs with weight-loss programs.

Q. Can you explain more about this weight-loss program?

A. The fat-loss program used by Dr. Kaats and his colleagues appears to be very effective. Health professionals have for years been encouraging people to increase their intake of dietary fiber. Fiber provides bulk, which helps to satisfy hunger, especially when food intake is reduced. Fiber may also slow the absorption of sugars and fats from the diet, which should trigger a weaker insulin response.

Carnitine, like picolinate, is an amino acid (a building block of protein). Carnitine is absolutely essential for moving fats into the mitochondria, the furnaces of the cells, where the fats are burned and energy is released. The mitochondrion is the only part of the cell where fat can be broken down into energy. Carnitine, just like picolinate, can be made in the body, so scientists squabble a lot about whether or not carnitine needs to be added to the diet. Muscles require a generous amount of carnitine to get all the needed fat into the mitochondria, so a supplement is wise for those who wish to lose fat and retain or develop muscle.

Dr. Kaats and his associates devised a plan that should, based on the clinical results, encourage fat loss and prevent muscle loss. Chromium picolinate plays a vital role in any program for fat reduction because it keeps insulin working properly. However, chromium is far more than an aid for fat reduction, so once you have reached your fat- or weight-loss goal, you should continue to take your chromium-picolinate supplements.

Q. Does chromium picolinate help to curb the appetite?

A. Chromium picolinate is not an appetite suppressant. However, its natural effect on insulin helps to keep you from going on snack-eating binges. From the moment insulin starts to become inefficient, control of the body composition becomes a problem. Body fat doesn't get used up the way it should, and cravings send people to the cookie jar or candy machine to load up on the fuel they think they need.

Our bodies have a built-in fuel gauge designed to signal when it's time to eat. This fuel gauge is a batch of specialized cells in the brain called the satiety center. These cells are critical in the regulation of body composition because they control hunger, stop insulin secretion, and cause excess calories to be burned. The satiety-center cells work by monitoring the amount of glucose available to the cells. The biological monitoring devices are inside the cells, so glucose must get inside in order to trigger any response.

Glucose uptake by the satiety cells is activated when insulin becomes attached to the cell receptors. By measuring the amount of glucose in these cells after insulin activation, the satiety center takes stock of both the glucose and insulin availability.

The satiety center is located in the area of the brain called the hypothalamus. The cells of the satiety center evaluate the input from the outside and orchestrate changes to help the whole body adjust. The cells in the satiety center communicate with cells capable of inducing hunger sensations. As long as glucose enters these cells, the command center detects an ample fuel supply, and the desire to eat is blocked. The fuel-monitoring cells are also connected to a communication network leading to the pancreatic cells. This network keeps the secretion of insulin from getting too high. Since insulin directs glucose into muscle and fat cells and away from brain cells, the command center helps to prevent fuel deprivation in the brain.

Q. How much exercise is needed to lose fat when taking chromium picolinate?

A. Exercise contributes to overall health and should become a part of everyone's life, but strenuous exercise is not necessary to help shed body fat when using chromium-picolinate supplements. Dr. Kaats and his associates conducted several studies with nonexercising people. In one double-blind study, the effect of two different quantities of chromium picolinate was compared by adding either the chromium or a placebo (inactive substance) to a liquid. The researchers gave the subjects no instructions about changing their diets, food intakes, or activity levels. They only asked the subjects to consume two drinks a day. At the completion of the seventy-two-day study, the group given the placebo showed no changes, while the chromium groups enjoyed astonishing changes.

The two groups given the chromium picolinate gained slightly more than 1 lb of lean body mass. The low-chromium-picolinate group (180 mcg of chromium as chromium picolinate per day) lost an average of 3.4 lb of body fat. However, the high-chromium-picolinate group (400 mcg of chromium per day) lost an average of 4.6 lb of body fat, or about 35-percent more. The average loss of body fat for all those taking chromium picolinate was 4.2 lb, with an accompanying increase in lean body mass of 1.4 lb. In contrast, the average fat loss of the people who took the placebo was only 0.3 lb! As expected, those taking the higher dose of chromium picolinate had the most dramatic changes in body composition, and older people (average age of fifty-five) showed better improvements than younger people (average age of thirty-six). This study was very informative because it showed that chromium-picolinate supplements helped to accelerate fat loss without exercise.

Q. Will chromium picolinate help everyone to lose fat?

A. Not everyone can get rid of excess body fat merely by taking chromium picolinate to make their insulin work more efficiently. Studies indicate that genetic factors can keep chromium supplements from having the desired results. However, if you wish to shed body fat, you should try a daily supplement of at least 400 mcg of chromium as chromium picolinate for one to three months. The risk, even financially, is negligible. If you do not experience any improvement in your body composition during this time, you should seek professional advice.

Q. Will exercise and chromium picolinate together help to increase the amount of fat loss?

A. Exercise and chromium picolinate are an effective combination for getting rid of body fat. Burning fat to produce body heat and to operate the basal metabolism uses about 75 percent of the energy derived from food. Muscular activity uses the remainder. Studies with exercising athletes have demonstrated that both men and women taking a chromium supplement lose more body fat than those taking a placebo.

Q. What is thermogenesis, and how is it affected by chromium picolinate?

A. Thermogenesis is the process the body uses to produce heat. The process only works when insulin functions normally, so chromium picolinate indirectly maintains thermogenesis.

The body cells have to maintain a constant temperature or they can't work correctly. If the temperature goes up (as in a fever), the biological machinery burns. If the temperature goes down, the machinery slows. An increase in temperature is detected by the brain, which in turn causes water to be secreted onto the surface of the skin (sweating) to evaporate and cool the body. Muscles and a special kind of fat cell called brown-adipose tissue keep the body warm. When the nerve cells detect a drop in the body temperature, they send an alarm to the brain. The brain then triggers the release of chemicals that prompt the cells to burn stored fat to produce heat.

In addition to keeping us warm, our muscles and

brown-adipose tissue are supposed to burn up any excess fuel we take in. If more than a predetermined amount of glucose flows into the monitoring cells after insulin has become attached, an alarm is sounded. Neurons in the brain send a message to the brown-adipose tissue and muscles to send fat to the mitochondria. According to some investigators, insulin resistance causes a retention of about 125 calories per day, which is why obesity is one sign of this disorder. Because chromium picolinate increases the efficiency of insulin, it reduces insulin resistance and helps to maintain thermogenesis.

Q. Does chromium picolinate help to increase the metabolism?

A. Chromium picolinate increases the pace of the body's metabolic activity because it keeps insulin working effectively. There are different ways the body uses energy, some of which you are not consciously aware. For example, whether you are completely at rest or moving a piano, your cells need some fuel to produce energy.

The unconscious goings-on are what keep your body alive. These goings-on coupled with the BMR burn about two-thirds of all the fuel you use in a day. The amount of energy you use just to keep up your BMR is surprisingly high. An average-sized man burns about 1,650 calories per day just to keep his body functioning. A woman uses about 1,500 calories per day. Since the BMR uses the major portion of the calories consumed, a reduction in this activity leads to a major reduction in calorie burning. The BMR is regulated in large part by the thyroid hormone known as triiodothyronine, or T_3 for short. Diabetes causes a decrease in the production of T_3, but proper treatment with insulin restores the production of this hormone to near normal. In other words, insulin has a profound influence upon metabolism because of its effect on the production of T_3, the hormone that stimulates the BMR.

4.

Chromium Picolinate and Cholesterol

Chromium-picolinate supplements help to control the type of cholesterol your body produces, as well as how much it produces. Chromium picolinate keeps insulin working efficiently, which in turn helps to keep glucose and fat from being turned into harmful cholesterol.

Q. Does chromium picolinate help to control cholesterol?

A. Since 1989, when it was first introduced, chromium picolinate has been shown to help control blood-cholesterol levels in several studies using humans and animals. In the first published study with humans, done at Mercy Hospital in San Diego, twenty eight volunteers with abnormally high blood-cholesterol levels were given either a placebo or 200 mcg of chromium as picolinate daily for forty-two days, followed by no supplementation for fourteen days. Each of the volunteers then became his or her own control by taking the substance not used during the first trial period. Blood was drawn and analyzed at the beginning of the study and then at the end of each of the forty-two-day trial periods.

During the period the volunteers took the chromium picolinate, the total cholesterol and LDL ("bad") cholesterol decreased. The total cholesterol decreased by 7 percent, while the LDL cholesterol decreased by 10.5 percent. During the final trial period, 22 of the volunteers had lower total-cholesterol levels, 2 had unchanged levels, and the remaining 4 had slightly elevated levels. In addition, 20 of the volunteers had decreased LDL levels, 3 had unchanged levels, and the remaining 5 had slightly elevated levels. The amount of HDL ("good") cholesterol increased slightly while the volunteers took the chromium picolinate. Absolutely nothing happened to any of the cholesterol levels when the volunteers took the placebo.

In a study of 180 type-II diabetics, Dr. Richard Anderson and his colleagues at the USDA observed a 15-percent decrease in total cholesterol when people were given 1,000 mcg of chromium as picolinate daily. In addition, animal scientists have seen some dramatic changes in cholesterol when chromium picolinate was added to feed.

Q. What does chromium picolinate do to LDL cholesterol?

A. Chromium-picolinate supplements cause a decrease in total cholesterol and LDL cholesterol. During the last couple of decades, you have probably been hearing about "good" cholesterol and "bad" cholesterol, which makes it sound like there are two kinds of cholesterol. Actually, there is only one kind of cholesterol, but it can combine with two different kinds of protein.

Because cholesterol is a fat, it cannot dissolve in watery fluids, such as the blood, so it has to be transported in the blood by proteins. The kind of protein to which the cholesterol becomes attached determines if it's good cholesterol or bad cholesterol. Apolipoprotein B, found in bad cholesterol, is particularly sensitive to chemical changes (oxidation) by renegade chemicals floating around in the body fluids. If apolipoprotein B becomes oxidized, or damaged, its properties change, and it becomes better able to enter the cells in the arteries and deposit cholesterol.

Studies of humans taking chromium-picolinate supplements have shown that the nutrient causes a decrease in apolipoprotein-B production. This indicates that chromium-picolinate supplements help signal the liver to cut back production of this cholesterol-transporting protein.

Q. Does chromium picolinate make the HDL-cholesterol level go up?

A. Chromium picolinate can increase the good cholesterol while decreasing the bad cholesterol. The other protein that carries cholesterol through the bloodstream is called apolipoprotein A1. Apolipoprotein A1 actually removes cholesterol already deposited in the blood vessels. When people use chromium-picolinate supplements, apolipoprotein-A1 levels increase. This is a biochemical signal that something beneficial is happening in the body. More apolipoprotein A1 is needed because the more cholesterol that is removed from the arteries, the better. Many cardiologists claim that an increase in apolipoprotein A1 is more important to health than a decrease in total blood cholesterol.

Q. How does chromium picolinate help to control cholesterol?

A. Chromium picolinate helps to control cholesterol simply by making insulin work efficiently. Insulin controls the body's use of fat as well as its use of glucose. High blood-insulin levels result in a lot of fat being released from the proteins that carry it through the bloodstream. A lot of that fat enters the adipose cells, but a good share is also taken up by the liver. This starts an unhealthy cycle.

The liver is very efficient at dismantling unwanted chemicals. All that fat entering it is not necessary, so the liver produces enzymes that break the fat into small pieces. These small pieces of fat can be used to make cholesterol, which the liver does in increasing amounts. To enable the newly formed cholesterol to enter the bloodstream, the liver then packages it with fatty acids and a certain kind of protein. The cholesterol therefore becomes LDL cholesterol. LDL cholesterol is very sensitive to attack by chemicals in the blood called oxidants. These oxidants change the protein, and the protein, along with its cholesterol and fat load, ends up inside the cells that line the blood vessels. Eventually, the cells become bloated and block the flow of blood.

Chromium picolinate helps to decrease the cholesterol level by reducing the amount of insulin the body needs. A reduced insulin need means a reduced amount of insulin in the blood. Less insulin in the blood helps the cells that burn fat to take fat out of the blood. The lower amount of fat in the blood lessens the amount of fat that ends up in liver and is made into cholesterol.

5.

Chromium Picolinate and the Muscles

Insulin does not stimulate the growth of muscles, but it has a very important role in helping the muscles to develop and in keeping the muscles from wasting away. Chromium picolinate is a nutrient needed to keep insulin working effectively, so it has a role in keeping the muscles healthy and well-developed.

Q. How does chromium picolinate help to develop the muscles?

A. When athletes in training, clinical investigators, and animal-science investigators use chromium-picolinate supplements, they see positive results in muscle development as well as in fat loss. Muscle development requires four very basic materials—glucose, fat, amino acids, and a hormone to activate the systems that make muscle protein. The glucose and fat are used almost exclusively as fuel to produce energy within the muscle cells. The amino acids are essential to make the proteins to form the muscles. The anabolic hormone is needed to send signals to the cells' nuclei to provide blueprints for turning the amino acids into protein. A lot of research has been pointing to insulin being the factor that determines whether or not all of those materials reach the muscle cells when they're needed.

Q. So, exactly how do insulin and chromium affect the muscles?

A. Poor insulin activity slows muscle development and promotes fat deposition. When insulin doesn't function properly, the muscles don't get enough glucose, amino acids, or fat. Fat, the preferred fuel for muscle, remains stored inside adipose cells, which accumulate on your hips and buttocks. When muscle can't use fat for fuel to produce energy, it turns to glucose. But if the cells don't respond to insulin's call to open the gates, glucose can't be transported inside to be used for energy. When fat isn't readily released from the adipose cells, and glucose can't get out of the blood and into the muscles quickly and efficiently, the muscles are forced to convert amino acids into energy. Sometimes, the muscles are forced to disassemble their own proteins to obtain fuel for energy.

Chromium keeps insulin funtioning efficiently, so the muscle cells can use glucose and fat for energy and amino acids to make protein. The proper use of glucose, fat, and amino acids certainly contributes to accelerated muscle development, but there is also another very important factor involved—the androgen that stimulates the manufacture of muscle protein. When muscles are exercised regularly, the brain signals the release into the blood of testosterone, the most potent androgen. Androgens are hormones that stimulate the muscles to make more protein and grow.

Testosterone stimulates muscle-protein generation, but the amount of testosterone produced is limited. To stimulate muscle manufacture beyond the limits of testosterone production, a backup is needed. DHEA, which is produced in vast quantities in glands on the kidneys, can also stimulate the development of muscle. It isn't as potent as testosterone, but it is an androgen. Also, the body can readily convert DHEA to testosterone. Chromium restores insulin efficiency, which allows glucose clearance with less insulin. With less insulin in the blood, the synthesis of DHEA is increased, providing a testosterone backup. The improved rate of muscle development observed in humans and animals given chromium picolinate is due to a combination of the more efficient utilization of glucose and fat for energy and a greater production of DHEA, which provides an added hormonal stimulus for muscle growth.

Q. Can chromium picolinate be used to replace steroid hormones?

A. Chromium picolinate is not a steroid hormone, but it certainly can help to develop the muscles without the side effects associated with steroids. Body builders as well as other athletes work tirelessly to develop their muscles. All too often, however, their progress isn't as hoped, so they turn to synthetic anabolic steroids. This is unfortunate because anabolic steroids cause kidney problems, liver cancer, and heart disease. Furthermore, the use of synthetic anabolic steroids to accelerate muscle development is totally unnecessary, since the body is capable of making enough natural steroids to stimulate muscle development without the dangers of side effects. Once again, to accomplish this, the body's insulin has to work efficiently, and that's where chromium picolinate can help. Athletes should use chromium picolinate and let their bodies make the steroids.

Q. Can chromium picolinate help muscle weakness?

A. It may, at least in some cases, but the research in this area so far is limited to animals. To explain, Dr. H.C. Gurney, Jr., a veterinarian in Conifer, Colorado, found chromium picolinate to be beneficial in preventing and reversing muscle deterioration in dogs. In a three-year study, Dr. Gurney divided 167 lame dogs into four groups. Lame dogs were chosen because lameness results in muscle atrophy (breakdown). The dogs weighing less than 20 lb were given daily supplements of 100 mcg of chromium as picolinate; the dogs weighing 20 to 50 lb were given 200 mcg; and the dogs weighing over 50 lb were given 400 mcg. To determine the effectiveness of the treatment, the dog owners were asked to rate as better, same, or worse their dogs' ease of rising without assistance, their endurance, and their gait.

The 27 dogs with the most advanced degree of muscle atrophy showed the least improvement; they may have been too far gone. Of those 27, the 8 that did show improvement had been given chromium-picolinate supplements for forty-five to ninety days. Among the dogs with a lesser degree of atrophy, 71 of 104 improved within fifteen to thirty days of supplementation. In dogs that were obese and had lost the ability to get up from a resting position without assistance, 6 of 9 showed improvement after thirty to forty-five days of chromium-picolinate supplementation.

6.

Chromium Picolinate and Aging

Insulin affects many cells in the body, including some glands that produce chemicals that slow aging. As long as insulin is healthy, your cells stay healthy and less likely to deteriorate. Chromium picolinate keeps your insulin functioning normally, so it can help your body stay active and vibrant longer.

Q. What's the relationship between chromium, insulin, and aging?

A. Research dating back to the 1930s showed that caloric restriction increased the life span in laboratory animals. Experiments along these lines have generally found that reducing the caloric intake by one-third throughout life—but maintaining adequate levels of the vitamins and minerals—extends the life span by about one-third. Recent, ongoing studies with primates have confirmed this effect.

Caloric restriction—the restriction of carbohydrates, proteins, and fats—maintains lower and steadier levels of glucose and insulin. Because less food is consumed, less insulin is required. In the ongoing primate studies, caloric restriction has also been shown to increase the resistance to diabetes. Chromium's effect on insulin in normal people is somewhat like the effect of a calorie-restricted diet on insulin. Insulin performs its many jobs efficiently. In a sense, chromium picolinate offers some of the benefits of caloric restriction without actual caloric restriction.

Q. How does chromium picolinate slow aging?

A. Again, chromium picolinate makes insulin work more efficiently. By doing this, it reduces the glucose level in the blood. This is important because glucose spins off hazardous molecules called free radicals, and high glucose levels spin off large numbers of free radicals. Many experts now believe that free radicals accelerate the aging process by damaging the cells. In fact, researchers view diabetes, with its characteristic high glucose levels, as a model of accelerated aging. This is because diabetics develop many diseases earlier than nondiabetics. By improving the efficiency of insulin, and thus lowering the blood-glucose level, chromium picolinate can slow the aging process.

In addition, considerable scientific evidence indicates that the functional capacity of three glands—the hypothalamus, the pineal, and the thymus—plays an important role in keeping the rest of our body parts from aging. Deterioration in one of these vital glands promotes aging or the loss of youth-retaining characteristics in the other two. Each of these glands is affected by the action of insulin. Each gland is therefore subject to the damage inflicted by the lack of chromium.

Dr. Henry Schroeder demonstrated that chromium deprivation shortened the life spans of rats and mice. More recently, Dr. Gary Evans and his students extended the life spans of rats by adding chromium picolinate to their diets. The longer-living rats had less glucose and less insulin in their blood. The longer-living animals also had much lower blood levels of hemoglobin A1C, which indicates good diabetic control and normal aging. The rat experiments demonstrated that bioavailable chromium (chromium picolinate) increases insulin efficiency and is needed for the maintenance of youthful cell performance.

Q. How does chromium picolinate help to prevent osteoporosis?

A. Chromium picolinate helps to prevent and even possibly reverse osteoporosis in women by functioning in the production of a substitute for the estrogen lost during menopause. Over 10 million women are afflicted with the age-related loss in bone density called osteoporosis. Because calcium is lost through the urine, bones lose their density, become brittle, and crack easily. This is accompanied by a loss of height and what has come to be known as a dowager's hump.

Osteoporosis occurs in women after menopause due in large part to the decreased production of the female hormones. Estradiol is the primary female hormone, and it has a profound effect on bone production. When there isn't enough of the hormone to stimulate bone manufacture, calcium, the main building material of bone, simply gets filtered through the kidneys and ends up in the bladder. Osteoporosis is caused by a diminished production of the hormone estradiol.

Osteoporosis may also be linked to a diminished DHEA production. DHEA is made in a gland tucked inside a glob of protective fat on each kidney. Scientists began to suspect the importance of

DHEA when they discovered it is the most abundant steroid hormone in the blood. In women, DHEA can be converted into estradiol. However, there isn't enough DHEA in the blood of older women because most have inefficient insulin. Malfunctioning insulin leads to higher blood levels of insulin. Insulin turns off the DHEA-manufacturing process, so most women at menopause not only don't make estradiol, but can't make enough DHEA to make up for the shortage.

Q. So, chromium picolinate helps the body to use calcium?

A. At least one clinical study, led by Dr. Evans, has provided strong evidence that chromium-picolinate supplements can be used to treat and prevent the loss of calcium after menopause. Postmenopausal women were given a daily chromium-picolinate supplement containing 200 mcg of chromium. Before the women started taking the chromium picolinate, their DHEA and estradiol levels were comparable to those of most women aged forty to sixty. Their urinary calcium losses were about twice those found in women who have not yet reached menopause. After taking the chromium supplements for a month, the women's DHEA and estra-

diol blood levels increased to resemble the levels of
women aged thirty to thirty-five. The amount of calcium they excreted decreased by half. A month after
the women stopped taking the chromium picolinate, their DHEA and estradiol levels decreased
again and their urinary-calcium excretion doubled.

Ordinarily, osteoporosis is treated with estrogen
or a combination of estrogen and calcium supplements. Estrogen is not an ideal treatment because it
has been shown to increase the chances of certain
kinds of cancer. A more desirable method of treatment is a combination of chromium-picolinate and
calcium supplements. Chromium picolinate is not a
drug and is inexpensive, safe, and readily available
without a prescription.

7.

Chromium Picolinate Is a Safe Supplement

Although one or two studies have suggested that chromium-picolinate supplements may pose risks, far more studies have shown that they are both a safe and effective nutritional supplement.

Q. Is chromium picolinate safe?

A. Chromium picolinate has been thoroughly tested and shown to be a safe supplement for humans and animals. So far, all of the research has shown a large margin of safety between the effective dose and toxic dose. After chromium picolinate is absorbed and utilized, any excess chromium is excreted through the urine. Chromium from food and food supplements does not accumulate in the body. The picolinate is transferred to the liver and coupled with a chemical that inactivates and detoxifies it. It then is also excreted through the urine.

A Japanese scientist studied the long-term effect of consuming picolinate. Using rats, he found the chronic-toxicity level to be equivalent to a human adult consuming 52.5 gm (about 2 oz) of picolinate per day. A person taking a supplement with as much as 800 mcg of chromium as chromium picolinate would absorb less than 7.0 mg of picolinate. That's 0.007 gm, or less than 0.001 oz.

Furthermore, people who do not take any kind of supplement containing any form of picolinate normally excrete about 20 mg of picolinate a day. This means that the body makes about three times more picolinate than a person would obtain by taking a large amount of chromium picolinate.

Q. Does chromium picolinate cause any side effects?

A. Since chromium picolinate was first introduced into the food-supplement market in 1989, reports of a few adverse reactions have surfaced. Some people seem to develop a slight skin rash when they start taking chromium-picolinate supplements. The reason for this is totally unknown. It may be a reaction to another ingredient in the capsule or pill, or maybe even to the chromium picolinate itself. If a rash appears and persists, first try taking a different brand of chromium picolinate. If the rash continues to persist, stop using the supplement.

The other adverse reaction that has occasionally been reported is dizziness occurring an hour or two after taking a chromium-picolinate supplement. This symptom occurs in both type-I and type-II diabetics who don't monitor their blood glucose closely and decrease their medication accordingly. However, when this symptom occurs in an individual who is not using insulin or a medication to control the blood glucose, it's an indication of some other problem with the blood sugar. An individual who has these symptoms but is not diabetic may in fact have clinical hypoglycemia, the inability to make the hormone required to keep the blood-glucose level from dropping too low. Alternatively, some people may have extremely sensitive and efficient insulin, and supplemental chromium may actually be detrimental. Regardless of what causes the reaction to chromium picolinate, if you become light-headed consistently after taking the supplement, you should stop using it immediately.

Q. What about chromium picolinate and cancer?

A. Studies show that chromium picolinate is a safe supplement, and it certainly doesn't cause cancer. One highly controversial study, done by researchers at Dartmouth College and George Washington University, claimed that chromium picolinate caused chromosome damage in hamster ovary cells grown in test tubes. The scientists who did the study used an amount of chromium that would be equivalent to a human taking daily supplements of 600,000 mcg of chromium as chromium picolinate. That's 1,500 to 3,000 times the daily recommended dose of chromium as picolinate. Despite the claims based on these questionable test-tube experiments, there is no evidence that chromium picolinate is toxic when taken as an oral supplement.

A number of years ago, Bruce Ames, Ph.D., of the University of California, Berkeley, devised a very effective method for testing chemicals that might cause cancer. In this method, known as the Ames test, the chemical in question is added to five different types of bacteria. Bacteria reproduce very rapidly, so the addition of a cancer-causing chemical to their food shows very obvious changes in their offspring. When changes are noted, the chemical is said to test positive and must be subjected to further tests. Biodevelopment Laboratories, an independent laboratory in Cambridge, Massachusetts, tested chromium picolinate using the Ames test. The supplement tested negative, indicating that it does not cause cancer.

Conclusion

Chromium is a nutrient essential for life and health. All people need it, yet it is very difficult to obtain from the modern diet. This is because the soil levels of chromium are often poor, and processing removes the mineral from food (and usually doesn't add it back).

Although many different types of chromium supplements are sold, chromium picolinate is one form that the body uses very efficiently. Chromium's most important role is in assisting insulin, a hormone that strongly influences how your body burns food—sugars and fats—for energy. Because chromium picolinate improves the efficiency of insulin, and most food-burning occurs in the muscle cells, chromium-picolinate supplements may contribute to better body composition.

Many multimineral supplements already contain chromium in the form of chromium picolinate. If you aren't already using a multimineral supplement that supplies at least 200 to 400 mcg of chromium as chromium picolinate a day, you might consider adding a little more. If your cholesterol is elevated, chromium picolinate may reduce it. If you feel tired after eating sugary meals, chromium picolinate may help your body to deal better with such foods.

Chromium, in the form of chromium picolinate, is a remarkable mineral whose fundamental roles in health were overlooked for years. Today, it's a popular supplement—popular because it has changed the lives of so many people for the better.

Glossary

Basal metabolic rate (BMR). The unconscious processes, such as breathing, that keep the body alive. The BMR uses most of the calories obtained through the diet.

Calorie. The basic unit used to measure the energy content of food. Specifically, 1,000 calories equal 1 kilocalorie, or Calorie. This book refers to Calories as calories.

Chelator. Chemicals with which metals combine for assistance in moving into and through the bloodstream. Picolinate is a chelator for chromium.

Cholesterol. A fatty substance used by the body to build cell walls and to create necessary chemicals. Cholesterol cannot dissolve in water, so it must combine with a protein (lipoprotein) and form either HDL cholesterol or LDL cholesterol in order to circulate in the bloodstream.

Cofactor. A substance that helps a protein to properly perform its function. Chromium is a cofactor of insulin.

Dehydroepiandrosterone (DHEA). A hormone that serves several functions in the body. It can be converted into testosterone for the purpose of building muscles. It can also be converted into estrogen for the purpose of preventing the loss of calcium through the urine.

Diabetes. The presence of glucose in the urine, a sign that the body can no longer control its use of the substance.

Glucose. The simple sugar used by the body as its basic fuel. Also called blood sugar.

Hormone. A chemical produced in a gland and sent through the blood to signal specific cells that they need to perform a function to keep the body working properly.

Insulin. The hormone that regulates the body's use of glucose, fat, and amino acids.

Testosterone. The primary male hormone, which has several functions in the body. One of those functions is the building of muscle.

Thermogenesis. The production of heat by the body through the burning of excess glucose or fat.

References

Anderson RA, Kozlovsky AS, "Chromium intake, absorption and excretion of subjects consuming self-selected diets," *American Journal of Clinical Nutrition* 41 (1985):1177–1183.

Anderson RA, "Chromium metabolism and its role in disease processes in man," *Clinical Physiology and Biochemistry* 4 (1986):31–41.

Anderson RA, Cheng N, Bryden N, Polansky MM, "Beneficial effects of chromium for people with type II diabetes," *Diabetes* 46 (1997):1786–1791.

Anderson RA, Cheng N, Bryden N, Polansky MM, "Lack of toxicity of chromium chloride and chromium picolinate in rats," *Journal of the American College of Nutrition* 16 (1997):273–279.

Broadhurst L, Schmidt WF, Reeves JB, Polansky MM, Gautschi K, Anderson RA, "Characterization and structure by NMR and FTIR spectroscopy, and molecular modeling of chromium (III) picolinate and nicotinate complexes utilized for nutritional supplementation," *Journal of Inorganic Biochemistry* 66 (1997):119–130.

Cefalu WT, Bell-Farrow AD, Wang ZQ, "The effect of chromium supplementation on carbohydrate metabolism and body fat distribution," *Diabetes* 46, Suppl 1 (1997): 55A.

Evans GW, Meyer LK, "Life span is increased in rats supplemented with a chromium-pyridine 2 carboxylate complex," *Advances in Scientific Research* 1 (1994):19–23.

Evans GW, Swenson G, Walters K, "Chromium picolinate decreases calcium excretion and increases dehydroepiandrosterone (DHEA) in post menopausal women," *FASEB Journal* 9 (1995):525.

Evans GW, "The role of picolinate in metal metabolism," *Life Chemistry Reports* 1 (1982):57–67.

Evock-Clover CM, Anderson RA, Steele NC, "Dietary chromium supplementation with or without somatotropin treatment alters serum hormones and metabolites in growing pigs without affecting growth performance," *Journal of Nutrition* 123 (1993):1504–1512.

Gurney HC Jr, "Muscle atrophy—the chromium connection," *Journal of the American Holistic Veterinary Medical Association* 9 (1990):5–6.

Hasten DL, Rome EP, Franks BD, Hegsted M, "Effects of chromium picolinate on beginning weight training students," *International Journal of Sport Nutrition* 2 (1992):343–350.

Jovanovic-Peterson L, Gutierrez M, Peterson CM, "Chromium supplementation for gestational diabetic women improves glucose tolerance and decreases hyperinsulinemia," *Journal of the American College of Nutrition* 14 (1995):530.

Kaats GR, Blum K, Fisher JA, Adelman JA, "Effects of chromium picolinate suppplementation on body composition: a randomized double blind placebo controlled study in different age groups," *Current Therapeutic Research* 57 (1996):747–756.

Kaats GR, Wise JA, Blum K, Morin RJ, Adelman JA, Craig J, Croft HA, "The short-term therapeutic efficacy of treating obesity with a plan of improved nutrition and moderate calorie restriction," *Current Therapeutic Research* 51 (1992):261–274.

Lindemann MD, Wood CM, Harper AF, Kornegay ET, Anderson, RA, "Dietary chromium picolinate additions improve gain, feed and carcass characteristics in growing-finishing pigs and increase litter size in reproducing sows," *Journal of Animal Science* 73 (1995):457–465.

McCarty MF, "The case for supplemental chromium and a survey of clinical studies with chromium picolinate," *Journal of Applied Nutrition* 43 (1991):58–66.

Page TG, Southern LL, Ward TL, Thompson DL Jr, "Effect of chromium picolinate on growth and serum and carcass traits of growing-finishing pigs," *Journal of Animal Science* 71 (1993):656–662.

Press RI, Geller J, Evans GW, "The effect of chromium picolinate on serum cholesterol and apolipoprotein fractions in human subjects," *Western Journal of Medicine* 152 (1990):41–45.

Schroeder HA, "The role of chromium in mammalian nutrition," *American Journal of Clinical Nutrition* 21 (1968):230–244.

Suggested Readings

Evans G. *Chromium Picolinate: Everything You Need To Know.* Garden City Park: Avery Publishing Group, 1996.

Fisher JA. *The Chromium Program.* New York: Harper Mass Market Paperbacks, 1996.

Passwater RA. *Chromium Picolinate.* New Canaan, CT: Keats Publishing, 1992.

Index